Relaxed or Natural ~

You Can Have Beautiful, Healthy, Black Hair

Guide to Growing Your Hair stronger, longer and healthier

Relaxed or Natural ~ You Can Have Beautiful, Healthy, Black Hair

Eddie Lee

ISBN: 978-1-4357-0398-8

Introduction

After experiencing a devastating allergic reaction to bonding glue and losing a tremendous amount of hair, I became incessant with finding methods to not only grow my hair back, but to achieve hair healthier than I had ever had. After 12 years of research I have compiled all of my findings relevant to helping Black women accomplish long, strong, healthy hair. This comprehensive guide to reaching your hair's fullest potential will tell you everything you need to achieve the hair you have always dreamed of.

In this book you will learn what ingredients are best for Black hair, as well as how to effectively care for relaxed and natural hair. You will learn how to most effectively care for braid extensions, minimize split ends, the correct way to wash and condition your hair and much, much more. This book is entertaining as well as informative. You will find yourself laughing while becoming equipped with everything you need to know to have beautiful, healthy, black hair.

****INCLUDES AN INGREDIENT GLOSSARY****

Contents

Introduction: *In the Beginning*   *1*

Importance of Moisure: *Remembering the Jherri Curl*   *5*

Importance of Protein: *Got Strong Hair*   *10*

Are Natural Ingredients Better: *I say... YES!*   *12*

Uh...Not In My Moisturizer: *Harmful ingredients in your moisturizer* *16*

Safe Ingredients in a Moisturizer: *Your hair will thank you*   *18*

How to Effectively Apply Moisturizer: *Probably not how you think* *20*

Damage of the Weave: *Bonding glue is not your friend*   *21*

Shampoos: *Don't just grab any one off of the shelf*   *24*

Conditioners: *Don't just put 'em in and wash 'em out*   *27*

Healthy Diet & Vitamins: *Is your diet healthy enough for your hair* *29*

Relaxing: *Doesn't have to be so damaging*   *32*

To Relax or Not To Relax, That Is the Question: To Preteens...NOT *40*

Healthy Ends: *Keep 'em moisturized to keep 'em longer*   *43*

Braid Extensions: *They need love too*   *49*

I Like Wearing Weaves: *That's fine as long as you take care of it* *53*

My Natural Story: *I decided to go natural because...*   *56*

Washing & Conditioning Natural Hair: *There is a difference*   *63*

Styling My Natural Hair: *My first attempt*   *65*

Pick Your Hair Care Products Wisely: *Overview of Ingredients*   *67*

Sweet Nature by Eddie Healthy Hair Care Products   *69*

Vitamins & Mineral: *Function and food supply*   *72*

Homemade Deep Conditioners: *Just open your refrigerator*   75

Helpful Tips: *More hair secrets revealed*   77

2-Strand Twist & Coil Instructions: *Learn the basics*   79

In The Beginning
(How I embarked on this hair journey)

When I was a little girl I remember having this reoccurring dream of having long flowing hair that would graze my waistline. In the dream, my hair always started out very short and then would spontaneously sprout out of my head until it reached my waist. I would go to school the next day and all the other little Black girls were so jealous; they would point at me and say my hair was fake. I would then let them feel it, just to prove to them that it was all mines. They lined up all around the playground in admiration and stood in line waiting for their turn to touch it.

As I got older I stopped having this dream. I think it was because I realized it was foolish to think that one day I, a full blooded Black girl, could ever have hair that would pass my shoulders, let alone graze my waistline. But, that didn't stop me from wanting the hair. I was in awe of the Black girls that had hair past their shoulders and downright jealous of the few I saw with hair to the middle of their backs. Like most of us, I assumed they had to have White somewhere in their ancestry or *"Indian in their family."*

Then when I was in the 6th grade this huge family moved across the street from me; there were five girls and two boys. Every single one of the charcoal little girls had beautiful long hair. Even the little boys had big thick cornrows down their backs. I immediately wanted to become their friend, with the hopes that some of their long hair would somehow rub off on me. I spent hours and hours playing in their hair, braiding and unbraiding, twisting and untwisting and brushing and combing. As I played with their hair, I would ask about the secrets to their phenomenal hair growth. None of them seemed to know why their hair was so long and contributed it to their mother's hair being really long; hereditary. That really left me hopeless because my mother's hair was even shorter than mines.

I can count on one hand the number of times I visited the beauty salon in my life. Growing up with a single, working mother, I had to take care of my own hair with little or no guidance. I can't recall when I started applying my own relaxer, but I'm pretty sure it was before the tender age of 13. As a matter of fact, I was relaxing, cutting and styling my peers' hair before then as well. In retrospect, I had no idea what I was doing. I was pretty much experimenting on these poor little unsuspecting children's heads. Fortunately, I never damaged anyone's hair so I didn't have to get a beat down.

As I grew older and faced many hair setbacks, including a few really bad short haircuts and a traumatic weave incident, I began to learn more about my hair and why it was having such a hard time reaching its full growth potential. Right before I decided to go natural I had grown, most of my hair longer and thicker than it had ever been before. Finally, my hair was past my shoulders and it didn't take me very long to get it there once I figured out the secrets. Now, I was getting compliments on how pretty, long and healthy looking *my* hair had become.

My mission was to grow my hair to the middle of my back. After achieving my initial goal, I knew there was no stopping me. I had learned the importance of protein and moisture balance, trimming my ends, minimizing heat usage, locking in moisture, baggying, relaxer stretching, a healthy diet, using the correct shampoos and conditioners, choosing good products, protective styling, supplemental vitamins, and a few other tricks I will share with you in this book.

Of course once I decided to go natural, I had to cut off all of my relaxed hair, which, like I said, had grown longer and healthier than it had ever been in my lifetime. Although it wasn't the easiest decision I had to make, it wasn't the hardest either. Once the possibility of growing long healthy hair had been realized, I knew that I could reach it again, and this time with even healthier hair. Exactly 18 months after cutting all of my hair off, it was back to the precut length, with no chemicals and no heat damage. Within two years my hair had reached my bra strap and only 2 inches from the middle of my back. Wow, my dream was materializing.

Importance of Moisture
(Remembering the Jherri Curl)

I remember going over my father's house when I was about 9 or 10 years old and seeing my stepsister with a fresh new Jherri Curl. I was amazed by her beautiful shiny new tresses; I wanted some of my own. It could have been my imagination, but I felt as if she was taunting me all weekend with her new look. It seemed that every time her name was called, she snapped her neck and slung her head as hard as possible so that the curls would swing from side to side and bounce all over the place. I wanted those curls so bad that I begged my father to put one in my hair right then and there. He said he had to talk to my mother when he dropped me off the next morning.

During the entire ride home, all I could do was imagine how beautiful my hair was going to look once I got that curl. I was so excited to get home that I practically jumped out of the car while it was still in motion. I ran up to the porch, where my mother was sitting, sipping lemonade. Partially out of breath from all the adrenaline pumping through my veins, I could barely speak. "Momma, I want to get a Jherri Curl like Monica's", I yelled. My father was standing behind me and further explained what I was asking of her and why. After my father finished his plea, my mother looked at both of us and said, "No." I was so devastated.

What was I going to do? I just had to find a way to get those bouncy, swingy curls.

The following weekend while visiting my father again, I felt the Jherri Curl envy wail up in me the minute I saw Monica's hair. So, I asked my father again if he would convince my mother to let me get one. Later that same day, my stepmother came home with a Jherri Curl kit and gave me my first official Jherri Curl. The process was long and the smell was awful, but after I saw the end result, it was worth it. My hair was gorgeous. My curls were even longer and prettier than Monica's. Now anytime *my* name was called, I snapped my neck and swung my hair too. I could finally feel those bouncy, swingy curls instead of just gazing at them.

I wore my Jherri Curl proudly; I loved it and I looked good. My hair grew to lengths it had never reached before. Within a year my hair was lying on my shoulders. Unfortunately this meant that all of my shirts were soiled by the constant supply of curl activator and moisturizer I had in it. I was beginning to experience break-outs on my pre-adolescent skin. I also encountered problems when I unexpectedly stayed the night over someone's house and I did not have one of those plastic Jherri Curl caps; no one wanted Jherri Curl juices all over their pillowcases or sofas.

As time went on and the novelty of swinging my hair until I almost had to be hospitalized for whiplash, experiencing hair to my shoulders, and comparing how much longer my hair was than Monica's, wore off, I realized that the curl was more of an inconvenience than anything. Besides, a lot of people started to convert to a relaxer and I figured it was probably time for me to get one and ditch the curl too.

When I decided to get a relaxer my mother was warned not to just put it on top of my curl. Instead of transitioning overtime, my mother decided to do the Jherri Curl process, but skip the curling rod part so that my hair could be straight. What a mistake! My hair was bone straight and when I tried to curl it with the curling iron, the curl wouldn't hold. Of course, I kept trying to curl it anyways because I wanted to wear it down. The constant heat of the curling iron gradually burned it out. My hair was so damaged and all I could do with it was pull it back into a ponytail; all that hair, literally, down the drain.

Did you ever have a Jherri Curl? It's okay, you can admit it; a lot of us did. If so, did you experience unprecedented hair growth? Let me explain why: All human hair, no matter your racial background is made up of the same thing. There is no chemical difference in the makeup of African-American hair in comparison with any other hair type. It has a cuticle (the outer layer), a cortex (the middle layer, composed primarily of keratin and moisture, plus melanin, which gives our hair its color), and a medulla (the center of the hair shaft). The only difference is the way the components are put together or the way they are structured.

Though there are exceptions, Black hair is usually more coarsely textured, tighter in curl pattern and more delicate and susceptible to damage from chemical treatments. The structure of Black hair can cause it to be more prone to breakage and excessive dryness. African-American hair is generally kinkier and more coily than other races, thus making it more difficult for the oil, sebum, which is secreted from the scalp, to reach the ends of the hair.

Sebum coats the hair and keeps it moisturized and healthy. The longer a person's hair gets, obviously, the further away the ends will be from the scalp, making it harder for the sebum to reach the ends. Have you ever noticed that hair seems to grow a lot faster when it is shorter and appears a lot healthier? This is because shorter hair is closer to the scalp, making it easier for the sebum to coat the entire strand, thus keeping the hair moisturized, which prevents breakage. Because the hair isn't breaking, it appears to be growing faster, but it's not.

Does your hair seem to always get to a certain length then just stops growing? Well, if you are still getting new growth every month, your hair is growing, but breaking off at the ends, which is usually caused by dryness. This is why people with Jherri Curls experienced extraordinary hair growth. Individuals with Jherri Curls constantly moisturize their hair. Those plastic caps serve two purposes: one is to prevent that goop from getting all over the place and the second purpose is to keep the hair moisturized at all times. A person with a Jherri Curl moisturizes their hair on a daily basis; some even moisturize more than once a day. This constant moisturizing helps minimize split end and allow the individual to retain more length.

I am not suggesting that you carry a bottle of activator or jar of moisturizer around with you, but I would suggest moisturizing the hair every day or at least every other day. Moisturizing doesn't mean slathering on a heaping handful of product, but letting your hair experience some sort of water based moisturizer, even if it's plain old water. It is important to make sure that at least the last 2-3 inches of hair is well moisturized in order to avoid excessive split ends.

Importance of Protein
(Got Strong Hair?)

Moisturizers keep the hair from becoming too dry and breaking off as well as gives it flexibility. Protein keeps the hair strong and regular use of certain proteins can actually thicken the hair. There are many different types of proteins. Some are extremely potent and should be used sparingly and cautiously.

These are the ones for extremely damaged and dry hair; hair that has been chemically processed, double processed or that is experiencing excessive breakage and shedding. These proteins are so strong that they stop the shedding immediately and results are typically noticed after the first use. Generally these kinds of protein treatments are so strong; they should only be used every 6-8 weeks or less.

There are also proteins that aid in thickening and strengthening the hair, but can be applied more often because they are not as strong; these are the proteins known as reconstructors. These proteins do not have a dramatic immediate effect, but overall hair improvement will gradually be noticed with regular use. These can be applied more often; every 4-6 weeks.

Finally, there are the mild proteins that are found in the majority of deep conditioner, slippage conditioners and some hair creams and oils.

These proteins are safe enough for regular use, but may cause the hair to become dry and brittle with overuse. When using them, or any proteins, it is extremely important to follow up with a good moisturizing regimen. If your hair creams or lotions have protein in them, you may want to add some jojoba oil, olive oil, or coconut oil to them to increase moisture and avoid potential over drying. If at all possible, stay away from hair creams or dressings that contain any kind of protein for this reason. Just remember that a good deep conditioner contains some sort of protein, but it is unnecessary in hair dresses or moisturizers.

Some of you may be saying, "I do moisturize my hair, I grease my scalp and I use *SuperDuperGrower* every day." Many products on the market today contain ingredients that cause more harm to our hair than good. Despite being called a moisturizer, they actually dry the hair out. Just because a product is expensive does not mean that it works any better than a less expensive one. The key is the ingredients in the *"Grow my hair down to my waist if I use this every day or your money back guaranteed"* hair grease. I have included a list of ingredients to stay away from, as well as ingredients to look for when you are purchasing a moisturizer.

Are Natural Ingredients Better?
(I Say…YES!)

One day while I was at the mall, I ran into one of the girls that lived across the street from me when I was a child. I instantly noticed how short and damaged her hair was. I couldn't believe this was the same head of hair I was in awe of when we were children. My hair was leaps and bounds healthier and longer than hers. As I finished up my conversation with her, I thought about all of the little girls that I've known over my lifetime that started out with a lot of hair and either lost it due to damage and breakage, or their hair seemed to just stop growing all together.

My own daughter was born with very little hair and then lost the little she had to eczema. She was left with a couple of strands of hair in the very top of her head, but other than that she was as bald as her bottom everywhere else. I was born with a head full of thick curly black hair and I assumed my daughter's hair would be the same, so this was hard for me to accept. I needed to find hair care products that were gentle enough for my daughter's delicate scalp yet effective enough to manage and strengthen my relaxed hair.

While visiting with my friend, I had noticed that her daughter's hair seemed to be thick and growing steadily. Her daughter was only a month older than mines, so I figured what she was using would work for my daughter as well. She gave me the name of a product and of course I rushed out to the nearest beauty supply store to purchase it. When I got to the store I was disappointed with how small the jar was and how expensive it was, but even more disappointed when I read the ingredients; it was full of everything I was told not to use, so of course I didn't purchase it, so I was back to square one.

After searching tirelessly, I decided to formulate my own hair care products made of all the healthy ingredients I had read about. The natural ingredients did the trick of not only growing her hair, but completely ridding her of eczema and fixing my hair problems as well. Soon, not only did her hair begin to grow; it began to thicken up and past the other little girl's hair by double the length; then triple. Within only two years, my daughter's hair had reached the middle of her back while the other little girl's hair seemed to remain the exact same length. After conducting a few surveys and further research, I concluded that overtime the mineral oil, petrolatum, paraffin and all of the other ingredients really does gradually stunt hair growth.

In my hair care workshops, I tell this story and each time I would have someone comment that when they were younger they used the "grease" products and they had long hair or that for years their grandmother pressed their hair using these products and they never experienced problems. (Of course just about every one of them were at the workshop because they were having issues growing their hair; so just by that my findings were somewhat confirmed) I would point out to them that maybe they didn't know their growth was stunted because they had never experienced the full growing potential that using natural products could give them; maybe they had accepted that ten inches of hair was as long as their hair would grow; not knowing they were depriving themselves of fifteen inches.

Some people are actually more sensitive to these ingredients and suffer more severe and rapid hair destruction, and some could go for years with slight and gradual hair lost, but either way, the fact is these ingredients are not healthy for the hair, scalp or body. Some people are actually allergic to the ingredients, which may cause excessive drying, dandruff and may exacerbate existing issues such as eczema, psoriasis or acute dermatitis. In 2009, I cut eleven inches of hair off; leaving myself with about three inches of hair. I didn't even know I could grow eleven inches, let alone cut that much off and still have some left before I learned

how to take care of my hair.

Uh…Not in My Moisturizer
(Do not let these harmful ingredients near your hair)

Petrolatum, also known as petroleum jelly, is a mineral oil derivative used for its emollient properties in cosmetics. When I first learned this fact, I was on the search for a moisturizer without petrolatum and found it extremely difficult to find. 95% of the moisturizers I looked at not only contained the ingredient, but it was the main ingredient listed on the product, no matter if it was an expensive or an inexpensive brand.

Petrolatum has no nutrient value for the skin or hair and can interfere with the body's own natural moisturizing mechanism, leading to dryness and chapping. Petrolatum often generates the very conditions it claims to ease; dryness. Manufacturers use petrolatum because it is extremely inexpensive. The majority of hair care products geared towards African-Americans contain petrolatum as the key ingredient, which may be a major contributor to the slow or stunted hair growth and breakage.

Mineral oil (a petroleum product) and its by-products are also used as an emollient in skin and hair care products. Like petrolatum, mineral oil cannot be absorbed properly by the body and it is phototoxic, allergenic and it stops the skin from using its own moisture-producing capabilities. It is not good to use mineral oil or it derivatives in any cosmetics, but look on the back of any of your "moisturizers" and I can guarantee that this is either the first or second ingredient listed. Regular use of either mineral oil or petrolatum on the scalp can remove the sebum, causing even additional drying. A good moisturizer should be water based. Here are a few other ingredients that a good moisturizer should NOT contain:

- Wax Ester - Spermaceti is sperm whale oil. (Banned in the US), but may be found in products from other countries.

- Hydrocarbon Oils & Waxes - Paraffin, Silicone Waxes, Ceresin, Silicone Oils, Ozokerite.

- Polyhydric Alcohol Esters - Propylene Glycol, Polyethylene Glycol (PEG), Sorbitan (Tweens), Mono and Di-Fatty Acid Esters of Ethylene Glycols, Polyoxyethylene Sorbitol, Propylene Glycol, Diethylene Glycol, and Polyethylene Glycol (PEG).

- Isopropyl alcohol

- Aluminum

- Parrafin – Mineral oil and petroleum product.

- Cocamide (DEA, DEA-CETYL phosphates, DEA OLETH-3 phosphates, Myristamide DEA, Stearamide MEA, Cocamide MEA, Lauramide MEA, Oleamide DEA, TEA-Lauryl Sulfate)

Here Are the Safe Ingredients
(Your hair will thank you)

Now, I know you are probably thinking, "Well, dang are there any ingredients I can use in my hair?" There are actually a lot of other ingredients that aid in excellent moisture balance and are healthy enough to not have any adverse side-effects. A good natural moisturizer contains essential fatty acids and herbs that trap in moisture and help to nourish the hair. It should help retain hydrations and shield the hair from environmental elements. Remember, the first ingredient should be water, followed by any of the following ingredients:

- Wax Esters - Beeswax, Lanolin (wool), Jojoba, Candelilla, Carnauba

- Steroid Alcohols - Lanolin, Alcohols, Cholesterol

- Fatty Alcohols - Cetyl, Stearyl, Oleyl, Lauryl Triglyceride Esters,

- Vegetable/African Butters - (Shea, Olive Butter, Avocado Butter)

- Phospholipids - Lecithin

- Polyhydric Alcohol Esters - Sorbitol, Glycerin, mannitol

- Fatty Alcohol, Ethers - Cetyl, Stearyl, Oleyl Hydrophilic

- Lanolin Derivatives - Natural Lanolin.

- Carrier Oils – (Grapeseed Oil, Wheat Germ Oil, Jojoba Oil)

Another way to keep your hair moisturized, especially in the summer time is by using humectants. Humectants adjust the exchange of moisture between the product and the air. They make it so the product can gradually release water, which aids in keeping the hair moisturized all day. Honey is a great humectant, and so is vegetable glycerin. You do have to be careful with using any humectants in the winter time, or in cold weather as the exchange also happens if the hair holds more humidity than the air. In this case, the air will take the moisture from your hair, leaving it dry. Generally, the best products for superior moisture and healthy hair are those that are water based and are not in a "grease-like" consistency.

How to Effectively Apply Moisturizer
(Probably not how you think)

Now that you know how important moisturizers are in aiding in hair growth and overall hair health, you need to know how to apply the moisturizer. Of course you know how to take the moisturizer out of the bottle or the jar and rub it into your hands and apply it to your hair, but believe it or not, some ways are more effective than others.

Many people apply moisturizers directly to the scalp. This practice is unnecessary; as the sebum is a natural moisturizer that already coats the scalp. If you have more than 5 inches of hair, it is important to make sure that you moisturize the last 2 inches of hair regularly, daily if possible. It is also a good idea to use a small amount of oil such as coconut oil or castor oil after moisturizing the ends to seal in the moisturizer. It is essential to apply moisturizer before you completely dry your hair, whether you use a blow dryer or let it air dry. Apply the moisturizer when the hair is approximately 70% dry so that you are allowing the moisturizer to infuse into the hair as it dries. Applying moisturizer on hair that is completely dry may cause the moisturizer to just sit on top of the hair.

The Damage of the WEAVE
(Bonding glue is not your friend)

About 11 years ago I went to the beauty shop, something I only did for very special occasions, to get a fancy up-do for a photo shoot. I went to one of the finest beauticians in my city because I didn't trust just anybody with my hair. I prepared to spend an entire day in the shop because I had to look my best. She relaxed my hair and then we decided that I would get a French Roll. In order to obtain the full, healthy looking French Roll I wanted, she had to add some hair. She did this by using bonding weave glue to adhere the weave to my scalp.

I left out of that salon feeling like a million bucks. This was my first official grown woman hairstyle, and I was looking super duper fly. After about 3 days, I started to experience an intense itching sensation that no amount of scratching could remedy. I was scratching with pencils, paper clips, hairpins, fingernail files, anything I could get my hands on. Finally I couldn't take the itching anymore so I decided to take the hair out. After recovering all the office and beauty supplies lost while scratching, I found that the bonding glue was so strong, I could have adhered my 2 year old son onto the top of my head with it.

I tried soaking my hair with conditioner for hours to massage the weave out, I tried piling on hair grease to slip it out; nothing worked.

Finally I called the beautician and she used some magical bond remover and my hair was free from the weave, but so damaged that my split-ends, had split-ends. I was horrified, but this was just the beginning.

As the week went on, my hair continued to itch. Not just a regular itch that a simple scratch could relieve, but an itch that seemed to be underneath my scalp. No matter how hard I scratched, I couldn't seem to satisfy the source of the itch. Even worse, upon each scratching session, I ended up pulling out a handful of hair. I can't remember how long I experienced the itch, but I do know that by the end, I had a bald spot in the crown of my head the size of a tennis ball. I also experienced mild to severe thinning in all of the areas the glue was applied. My hair was a mess and needless to say, I was traumatized.

After about a month or so, I started to feel stubble growing back, which gave me some hope. But then I noticed that the hairs seemed to be growing in much thinner. Some areas were not experiencing any growth whatsoever. The areas that did grow seemed to break right off with the slightest manipulation. After about 6 months, I had not achieved any significant growth, so I decided to seek some professional help. I went to a cosmetologist that said it was probably alopecia. I went to my own doctor who concluded the same thing and started me on steroid shots in the thinning and balding areas. This did no good. I went to a dermatologist who determined I had an allergic reaction to the glue and permanent damage to my hair follicles. Although all of them gave me a diagnosis, no one gave me a solution that actually worked.

This is when I decided to do some research. I had to grow my hair back. I was embarrassed, losing self confidence; my self-esteem was suffering, not to mention I looked like George Jefferson from behind whenever I let my hair out of the ponytail that was *trying* to disguise the bald spot. I got on the computer and researched any and every hair topic I could think of. I checked out every hair book from the library and read every Black hair care magazine I came across. It took me years to find the right combination of products and the best regimen for me to reach my own greatest hair growth and after years of research, I was able to realize my hair's fullest growth potential, which was a lot more than I had ever imagined.

Shampoos
(Didn't know they could be so dangerous)

When you wash your hair, does it seem really dry and brittle? Have you ever avoided washing your hair for weeks at a time, some of us for months, because you just knew it was going to take a few days for your hair to come back to life; to soften up or feel moisturized? Well, the reason for the excessive dryness is that washing the hair with certain shampoos strips it of all its moisture because of the "bad ingredients" the majority of shampoos contain. Further damage is actually being done to the hair if you "repeat" as the bottle suggests.

Approximately 90% of all shampoos contain Sodium Laureth Sulphate (SLES), and Sodium Lauryl Sulphates (SLS), which can be found in common household detergents such as dishwashing liquids, hand soap, washing powder, and many others. These ingredients function is to create foaming action. And to break down "grease, which is why it is also used in floor and engine degreasers. SLS and SLES may lead to deficient hair property, corroded hair follicles and inhibited hair growth, contributing to hair loss.

SLS and SLES are possibly two of the most dangerous ingredients in personal care products. According to American College of Toxicology, both SLE and SLES can cause malformation in children's eyes. Other research has indicated SLS may be damaging to the immune system, especially within the skin.

I know 90% is a huge number of shampoos that you must stay away from, but that still leave 10% and fortunately you only need one or two good ones. Any local health food store will have a wide variety of different shampoos you can use. Although many of these shampoos are sulfate free, they may not contain the added oils and moisturizers as Sweet Nature's Inspiration Shampoo does.

Now that you know the correct shampoos to use to benefit your hair's health, you no longer have an excuse to go more than a week without washing your hair. I know every week sounds like a lot to the women that are used to washing their hair on relaxer day only, but the benefits will far out way the small inconvenience. Water is our hair's best friend and many Black women who have realized this have started to wash their hair daily or every other day, resulting in healthier hair. Now, I'm not going to pretend that I am one of those women because I am not; I only wash my hair once a week. But, I do know that moisture is the number one component to growing black hair long, and all moisture is derived from water. Besides, washing the hair does not only cleanse the hair and scalp, but the massaging motion of washing the hair will stimulate circulation in the scalp, especially if you add a few drops of peppermint oil to your shampoo. It has been said that a stimulated scalp leads to healthier and longer hair. Just a reminder that even after finding the perfect shampoo, it is a good idea to either use a clarifying shampoo, which will cut through any build up or do an apple cider vinegar rinse or a baking soda rinse to clarify the scalp every 6-8 weeks and then go back to using your regular shampoo.

Conditioners
(Don't just put 'em in and then wash 'em out)

Each shampoo should be followed up with a deep conditioning. Conditioning is one of the essential steps that, if not executed correctly, may be the deciding factor in how much hair you retain. Instant conditioners, such as the *99 Cent Store* conditioners that pour out of the bottle slightly thicker than water will not suffice. They are used strictly for the "slippage" factor to aid in detangling. They do not penetrate the hair shaft. A deep conditioner will either state that it is a deep conditioner or a reconstructor; the directions will indicate that you should keep it in for approximately 15-20 minutes; or there will be an indication that applying heat will further the conditioning effects. No matter what the instructions read, always use a plastic cap with some sort of heat to process the conditioner, even if it's just body heat, otherwise, it's pretty much a waste.

Deep Conditioners and reconstructors are used for strengthening the hair. It is important to use a deep conditioner because they are able to penetrate the hair shaft and go inside of the strand instead of just sitting on the outside. Penetration takes approximately 15 minutes, which is why some deep conditioners suggest keeping it on for this amount of time. Also, heat can cause the shafts to open quicker than 15 minutes, but it's impossible to tell how much more quickly. Therefore, it is always wise to keep deep conditioners on for a minimum of 15 minutes. After it has processed, first detangle with your fingers and then with a wide tooth comb. Once the hair has been detangled, rinse the deep conditioner out and then do a flash rinse at the very end with water as cold as you can possibly stand it so that the hair cuticle will snap back closed.

Healthy Diet & Supplemental Vitamins
(Is your diet healthy enough for your hair)

Hair growth really depends on the span of your hairs' growth cycle, which can be anywhere from 2 to 6 years; genetics; and your overall health and diet. Unless a person is suffering from an excessive amount of stress for a prolonged period; illness, or maybe taking medication that either stunts the hair growth or makes the hair fall out, we are all experiencing hair growth at all times. Hair grows an average of .5" per month, give or take. When I say this, I don't mean White people's hair, but *all* types of hair. Yes, Black women have the potential to grow our hair as long as or longer than our White counterparts.

Although a person can do nothing about their heredity or the life span of their hair, we can all do something about our diets. It is very important to watch what we take into our bodies for our bodies' health, as well as the health of our hair. We also need to make sure our water intake is substantial. Before I embarked on my journey to mid-back length hair, I was a total sugar addict. I ate cookies for breakfast, ice cream for lunch, threw a few candy bars and licorice in for daily snacks and washed it all down with a tall cup of juice. I was a fast food queen and loved the fries at the golden arches and the double cheeseburgers too. Not only was this damaging to my body but it was also wreaking havoc on my hair.

Our hair needs nutrition from the inside out. Suitable nutrition is imperative for growth of hair follicles and healthy hair fiber. If your dietary intake is lacking in hair-friendly foods, all the expensive shampoos, conditioners and products you are spending your hard earned money on will produce minimal results. If you are anything like me, changing your diet will be extremely difficult. I gradually became conscious of labels, counting the grams of sugar; then the fat and sodium content. There was no way that I was going to give up all of my junk food cold turkey, so I either eliminated or decreased the bad ingredients gradually. Fortunately, the longer I did this the easier it was for me. My taste buds changed and my body could no longer withstand the continuous sugar assaults.

During my transition to better eating habits, which I am still undergoing after 10 years, I decided to take vitamins to supplement the nutrients I was missing in my diet. I started out taking a multi-vitamin and within a month or two, I began to notice my fingernails were healthier and stronger and I had a lot more energy. While shopping for my multi-vitamin, I came across vitamins that were specifically tailored towards growing healthy hair. I bought them and noticed results after taking the first bottle. My hair seemed thicker and my nails grew stronger and longer.

Over the years, I have changed to and from several different brands of hair vitamins. I do believe some are superior over others as some have fillers, are missing key vitamins, or have key vitamins in a very low dosage. Some of the hair vitamins also exclude minerals that aid in hair growth and health. I have included an easy chart at the end of the book to reference which vitamins and minerals aid in healthy hair growth as well as which foods contain these vitamins and minerals.

Relaxing
(Doesn't have to be so damaging)

For many years I surveyed the Black woman's relaxed hair. What I continuously found was that We suffered from extremely thin edges, see through and severely split ends, dry brittle looking hair, excessive breakage in the nape, and generally unhealthy looking hair. It was a rarity to see a Black woman with a head full of healthy hair. I'm sure if every one of these women could have healthier hair, they would. I know this because approximately 85% of all hair care products, including weaves and wigs, are purchased by Black women, yet we have the most damaged hair of all races.

The reason our relaxed hair continuous to be damaged and appears not to grow is because we have no idea of how to effectively take care of it. The assumed experts; the beauticians are suppose to be the main source of information for growing healthy hair, so we ask them for their advice and go to them to have them take care of our hair. Not to offend any beauticians, but a lot of them have no better idea of how to make our hair grow to its fullest potential than the average woman.

A lot of beauticians are probably not as candid as they could be as to the proper care and products used because they want to continue to be your primary source for your hair care needs, which is logical. I remember one beautician that would pour her hair products into unmarked bottles just so her clients couldn't go out and purchase the products. Even if they asked, she would not reveal the name brand. I am not a licensed cosmetologist, but I have years and years of research and experience with growing, relaxing and experimenting with Black hair and I have effectively grown my hair and others to unprecedented lengths. As well as grown people's hair that suffered from alopecia and Trichomania.

Let me give you a quick little science lesson. All hair that is curly is curly because the keratin proteins contain amino acids called cystienes. These cystienes link to each other by disulfide bonds; the more disulfide bonds, the curlier the hair. Relaxers simply break these disulfide bonds so that they cannot chemically reform. So, relaxers are permanent and cannot be removed without cutting the hair. The chemicals penetrate your hair shaft and break protein bonds inside, leaving curly hair limp (straight). The very outcome of the relaxing process is the result of partial hair destruction. Therefore, relaxed hair is, by definition, weaker than natural hair. Weaker hair means that the hair is more prone to breakage and becomes damaged much easier. Therefore, relaxed hair has to be given special attention.

The overall health of relaxed hair depends on how well it is taken care of before, during and after each touch up. One way to make sure that relaxed hair doesn't become too damaged is to never over-process when relaxing the hair. Always keep applications at or under the maximum instructed time. Another thing is to make sure that you do not double process the hair. Double processing is when you apply relaxer to portions of the hair that has already been relaxed; it is extremely important to touch up the new growth only. Double processing also occurs when hair is colored and relaxed in the same time period; wait 4 weeks before taking on a second process and make sure the hair is not overly damaged or experiencing excessive breakage. Many people do not know that braiding the hair with synthetic extensions shortly after a relaxer also constitutes double processing. This occurs because synthetic hair contains chemicals that cause further drying of colored or relaxed hair, making it more susceptible to breaking.

I know most women with relaxers love the super straight look, but it is much better to apply the relaxer for the minimum allotted time instead of trying to get the hair bone straight; this can cause limp lifeless and thin hair that is more prone to breakage. Today, many women are doing what is known as telaxing their hair. This is a cross between a relaxer and a texturizer. Telaxing is achieved when the relaxer is left on the hair for only half of the instructed time. The hair will not be totally straight, but it will maintain more thickness, body, strength and moisture. When you apply heat such as flat-irons or curlers to telaxed hair, it will look no different than relaxed hair, except it will likely appear fuller and healthier.

Telaxing is not an easy concept to grasp for everyone. Most women, who relax, do so to completely get rid of new growth and to have super straight hair. Because telaxing doesn't completely straighten the new growth and mostly loosens it, the outcome will be somewhat different then the relaxed hair, leaving the hair two semi-different textures if you have already relaxed in the past. Once a person sees the benefits of telaxing, some choose to slowly trim off the relaxed hair so that one day they will have a full head of telaxed hair, which will ultimately be fuller and healthier. Many women find that telaxed hair takes a little more time and effort to manage than relaxed hair, but is a lot easier to manage than completely natural hair. Before going totally natural, this is what I did to maintain thickness and overall health of my hair. Remember, no matter if you telax or relax your hair, be sure to use a protein rich deep conditioner to strengthen the hair and a great moisturizer regularly until the next process.

Another way to ensure a healthier head of relaxed hair is to relax your hair as seldom as possible. The least applications per year, the healthier your hair will be at the end of that year. I used to relax my hair every 4 weeks; approximately 12 relaxers a year; this is way too much. In general, we should wait until we have at least 1" of new growth before applying a touch up. On average a person grows a half inch of hair per month. So, at the very most, we should be relaxing our hair every 6-8 weeks; 6-8 relaxers a year. Why not challenge yourself and make it 3-4 per year.

Waiting longer than 4 weeks to relax my hair was one of the most difficult things I had to learn to do when my hair was relaxed. I absolutely hated new growth with a passion and the more new growth I had, the more my hair would break and shed. The breakage occurred because when our natural hair grows, most likely it has some level of curl or kink to it, and the relaxed hair, of course is straight, and where the two textures meet, "the line of demarcation", the hair becomes more fragile and prone to breakage if it is not given special attention.

During this stage, it is imperative to make sure the hair is moisturized daily. Hot oil treatments are an excellent idea during this time as well as making sure the hair is deep conditioned at least once a week.

Breakage will also be minimized if the hair is detangled with a wide-tooth comb while the conditioner is still in the hair. It would also be wise to apply a leave-in conditioner to aid in strengthening the hair. Remember to be extra gentle while combing the hair at this stage of the growth process. If possible, wash the hair in the shower (do not use hot water) or with the head backwards, in the way it is done at the beauty salon. This will cut down on tangles and the breakage detangling may cause. While you are washing the hair, gently finger comb it instead of rubbing it, which may cause tangling.

Many women understand the potential dangers a relaxer may cause, but they do not want to go natural for various reasons, so they stretch their relaxers. Stretching a relaxer is basically trying to get down to as few relaxer applications per year as possible. I know women who got down to relaxing their hair only twice or even once a year. I wasn't that zealous, but I was able to reach 10 weeks; cutting my applications down to less than half of my previous count. What made it easier for me was wearing low maintenance hair styles. Once I hit the 4 week mark, I would wear a roller set or maybe some cornrows for 2 weeks and then at week 6, I would get extensions for the remainder of the 10 weeks. Just remember when getting extensions, be very careful with not getting them put in too tightly. Extensions and braids that are too tight contribute to thinning edges and traction alopecia.

I was very fortunate because I was able to do all of the above styles myself and in the comfort of my own home. For those who are not so fortunate, there are an abundance of resources on the internet or in your public library that will provide tutorials on hundreds of different hair styles. I know many people who wear wigs or weaves during the harder times as well. Just remember not to neglect your own hair while in extensions, weaves, or wigs. Your hair still needs to be washed, deep conditioned, and moisturized regularly. If you do decide to use weave, please get it sewn in and DO NOT use bonding glue.

Today we have a choice to use lye or no lye relaxers. The lye relaxer is better for your hair because it doesn't leave it as dry and brittle as no-lye. But, a no lye relaxer is better for your scalp in the event the relaxer actually comes in contact with the skin; it will cause less burning and irritation. In the entire 20 years I used a relaxer, I have never used a lye relaxer because I have always applied my relaxers myself and I can't remember a time that I did not get some relaxer on my scalp. The key to countering the dryness and brittleness of the no-lye relaxer is to add extra virgin olive oil to the relaxer. It would also be beneficial to apply a reconstructor with keratin protein to your hair after each no-lye relaxer

application followed up by an extra moisturizing regimen.

To Relax or Not To Relax…
(If you are a preteen…The answer is Not!)

When I was about 10 years old or so, I got my first relaxer, so I am by no means condemning anyone who chooses to relax their hair. I believe that every person has a right to wear their hair however they see fit, but I also believe every person also has the right to know what their choices may be doing to their hair and bodies. As mentioned in the last section, relaxers are made with extremely strong and toxic chemicals and are formulated to obliterate the outer layer of the hair shaft or cuticle, thus causing the hair to be weaker.

As we age, it's a normal for the hair to be somewhat thinner and not as strong or grow as long, but if you have used a relaxer, chances are that by 40, you may experience more thinning and damage than someone who had not used a relaxer. Also remember that most people relax their hair as a pre-teen, so by the age of 40, many women have used relaxers for well over 25 years. This may lead to irreversible follicle and scalp damage as well as health issues.

Sodium Hydroxide is an extremely strong chemical used in some relaxers because it's effects are permanent and drastic. However, this same sodium hydroxide is found in drain cleaners which are primarily used to break down the hair that clogs the sink...which demonstrates the strength of this chemical. The majority of chemicals in relaxers are not safe for our skin, which is why it is recommended to use gloves when applying them. Yet, we apply these chemicals to our hair, which most of the times, inadvertently end up on our scalps. Preteens bodies and organs are not developed enough to be able to handle these toxic chemicals as well as an adults. Their follicles may not be mature enough to withstand the abuse and could begin to develop malformed hair; in some cases permanently.

Several studies have shown that, much like a birth control or nicotine patch, toxic chemicals from relaxers and other hair products may be absorbed through the scalp in sufficient enough amounts to increase the risks of adverse health effects in women and their unborn infants including, but not limited to premature births and low birthrates. A recent report shows that cosmetologist who regularly use hair chemicals are at higher risk for miscarriages.

Many of us relaxed our hair because it was the in thing to do, kind of like smoking was in the early days, but now, it's not so cool as we are finding that cigarettes account for an alarming amount of cancer cases. Like cigarettes, relaxers have several toxic chemicals that have been linked to cancer. I know that being natural isn't the easiest thing to do but I also know that it is important to be educated when it comes to putting things in our bodies that may be harmful.

Healthy Ends
(Keep 'em moisturized to keep 'em healthy)

Although at some point in time every person should trim their ends, there really is no set time frame to do it. Some people set a schedule such as every 6 weeks; some people wait until the ends look as if they need a trim; and, some people decide to set a length goal, pass it and then trim the hair back to that length. It really depends on the person's preference, but the need to trim is unavoidable. Split ends are caused by exposure to harsh weather, sun, and chemicals, lack of moisture or too much protein amongst other things. The ends have been around the longest, thus exposing them to more elements than the rest of the hair. In general, people with chemically treated hair may need to trim more often than those without, but there are definitely exceptions to this rule.

Getting my ends trimmed was the only reasons I patronized a beauty salon. When I was relaxed and learning about growing my hair, I continuously read about keeping the ends trimmed to promote healthy growth. I wanted to make sure I had an expert service my ends. Besides, I'm thinking if I tried to trim the back of my head, I would end up with a lopsided bob. At first, I got my ends trimmed every 4 weeks. After doing this for a few months, my beautician told me that I didn't need to come in that often because I wasn't getting any split ends, so I decided to go in every 6 weeks. Instead of getting my ends trimmed, I decided to just get them dusted, which is snipping the wild and unruly strands to make the hair look blunt and neat without getting a full trim. I had learned to take such good care of my ends that I very rarely needed an actual trim.

Now that I am natural, I trim my hair every 6-12 months, but I dust the ends between trims. I do not use any chemicals on my hair, I moisturize my hair each day and seal the ends with a heavy oil, I wear protective styles 90% of the time and I don't use any heat on my hair, so my ends aren't really at risk for a lot of damage. I am also one of the people that grow my hair to a certain length and then trim it, just because I have an ultimate hair goal of mid-back length. I grow my hair a little past each mini-goal and then trim it up to the mini-goal. This way I feel as if I am always on track with my ultimate goal. I'm pretty sure it's a psychological thing, but it makes me feel better.

Now, there is a debate regarding the necessity of trimming split ends. I have literally read hundreds of articles regarding this and I have seen both professionals and hair fanatics take a different stance on the subject. Some people swear that trimming split ends make the hair grow, while others explicitly renounce this theory, indicating that just because you trim off the end of a strand, doesn't make the strand suddenly begin to sprout out of your scalp, nor does it make your hair grow any faster. There is no physiological evidence that suggest trimming the hair makes any difference in the rate of growth or the thickness of the strand. Therefore, I have to agree with the latter.

Many people speculate that if we do not trim split ends, then the split will travel up the entire hair shaft causing the entire strand to be damaged or break at the scalp. Others insist that the hair will just break right off where it is weakest or split; therefore there is really no need to trim, if you take really good care of your hair, except to keep the hair looking neat. Honestly both theories make sense to me, but after testing it several times on my own hair, I notice that the hair does usually break where it's weakest. On many occasions, I've even tried to split the hair all the way up, but it would break off instead of ride upwards. Although my experiment has lead me to believe split ends usually break off eventually, I still prefer to trim them rather than letting them fall off.

No matter whom you are, at some point you will experience split ends. This is normal although somewhat upsetting and frustrating to some; there's no way to totally avoid them. But, there are definitely ways to minimize split ends and keep as much of your hard earned hair growth:

- Minimize heat usage; if at all possible, eliminate it.

- If you do have to use heat, use it on the lowest setting.

- Instead of blow drying, let your hair air dry 70-80%, moisturize and then flat iron it. This will not only eliminate the damaging blow dryer heat, but not allowing your hair to dry completely before flat-ironing will lock in moisture.

- If you do blow dry your hair, only blow dry it 70-80%, add moisturizer and then curl or flat-iron. This will lock in the moisture as well.

- Apply ice cold water to the ends of your hair before flat ironing or curling. This will close the cuticle and lock in moisture.

- Always use a heat protector when using *any* heating appliance.

- Keep your hair in protective styles. Protective styles are styles that "hide" your ends such as braids, buns, twist, cornrows, etc. It's also a good idea to find a style that does not allow the ends to rub directly onto clothes. Remember not to do any style too tight.

- After moisturizing the hair, seal the ends with heavy oil such as castor oil or coconut oil.

- Use the baggy method. Usually when using the baggy method, the hair is pulled back into a ponytail. Moisturizer is then applied to the ponytail and then the ponytail is covered with a plastic sandwich bag or you can improvise and use a piece of a plastic grocery bag, saran wrap, or a shower cap. Most people either secure a phony ponytail over the plastic or just wrap it with cloth; anything to make sure the plastic is not exposed. This will supply a constant source of moisture to your ends, like the Jherri Curl cap did for the entire head.

- Applying a leave-in conditioner after washing will also minimize breakage as it strengthens the hair.

- Stay away from brushes. I know you have probably heard that brushing your hair for 100 strokes will make your hair grow and shine. This is true for other races, but not for Blacks. Brushes pretty much tear the hair right out of our heads. If you must use a brush, use it sparingly and use a brush with boar bristles and not one with rubber or plastic ones.

- Stay away from combs with seams. The seams in the cheaply made combs cause damage because the seams snag on the hairs, causing them to tear. Never comb your hair with combs that come packaged 15 for $2. If you've already purchased these combs and don't want to discard them, you can file the seams down with a fingernail file and they will work just as well. But, if you don't want to do this, just read the package, many combs advertise the lack of seams right on the package.

- If you are natural, never comb your hair while it is dry. Moisture provides some slip for our coily hair and allows for a comb to get through easier than dry hair.

- If you are relaxed, never comb your hair while it is soaking wet. When relaxed hair is wet, it's at its longest point and putting extra stress on it with a comb will either cause it to stretch more, if it has a significant amount of elasticity, or to just break off if it doesn't.

- Sleep with a satin scarf or on a satin pillow to avoid the hair rubbing up against any rough materials while you are sleeping.

- When getting your ends trimmed, make sure that the shears are ultra sharp; dull shears contribute to split ends. Be sure that the shears have not been used to cut anything other than hair. If at all possible, invest in a professional pair of shears and request your beautician use yours so that you know the history of them.

These tips will not eliminate split ends all together, but they will definitely allow you to reach your goal a lot quicker.

Braid Extension
(They need love too)

When I resolved to go natural, I decided that braid extensions would be the easiest and most convenient way for me to grow my hair out as quickly as possible. Braid extensions are a great way of growing your hair because the ends are protected, there's very little maintenance involved, and therefore you are not using any combs or brushes, you also have great access to your scalp, giving you the ability to deliver massage it better, and for the products to deliver nutrients to the scalp more effectively; and the style last for weeks. But, if braids are not applied and taken care of properly, you will definitely do more damage than good.

Many people don't realize that braid extensions are coated with a chemical that causes the hair to dry out excessively. So, if you apply a relaxer and then immediately get extensions you are double processing your hair, causing it to become even weaker and more brittle, especially since the hair is already at its weakest point immediately following a relaxer. Therefore, you should wait two weeks after relaxing to get braid extensions.

One way to combat the excessive dryness from extensions is to soak the entire braid in apple cider vinegar for 15-30 minutes and then rinse with cool water before braiding. This will strip the chemical from the extension, thereby making it safer for the hair. Don't worry about the smell, it will go away before the hair is finished being braided.

It is essential to find a braider that understands that when you get your hair braided, you only want the hair braided and not your scalp. Too many times I sat in the braiding chair and allowed the braider to squeeze and pull my hair so tight that I felt like my scalp was on fire. Yet, I didn't say anything because I assumed that braids had to hurt to look neat and to stay in longer; this is a nasty myth. I remember spending $150 on braid extensions and taking them out in 3 days because my head hurt so badly. When I did take them out, my edges came right out with them and my scalp was sore for weeks.

It is important to know that getting braid extensions doesn't mean you don't have to do anything to your hair at all. Your hair still needs to be washed, deep conditioned and a leave-in conditioner needs to be applied weekly. The hair should also be moisturized regularly using a moisturizing spray.

Although you should stick to your regular regimen when you have braid extensions, you absolutely have to execute the regimen differently. Washing the hair should always be done in the shower using luke warm to cool water. After soaking the hair, you should pour a squirt of Sweet Nature by Eddie's shampoo in a cup and then fill the cup with cool water, add a teaspoon of baking soda or apple cider vinegar then pour directly onto the scalp. Massage the scalp only, being careful not to manipulate the braids. Now, mix the shampoo again and pour it through the braids, while gently squeezing the braids as you move down the length of the braid. Continue until all traces of shampoo are out of the hair. You can also pour the shampoo into a spray bottle and spray it directly onto the scalp and braids.

Next you need to deep condition the hair, but you do not want to apply it the same way you would apply it to your loose hair. Deep conditioners are generally thick, so this would be a great time to use one of the homemade deep conditioner recipes found in the back of this book because most of them are thin enough to be put into a spray bottle. Or, if you still want to use a deep conditioner, dilute it with water to a yogurt consistency so that it is not too thick to spray out of a sprayer. After filling the bottle, saturate your braids with the mixture and then put on a plastic cap, or you may need a plastic grocery bag if you tend to wear your extensions really long like I do. Your body heat should be enough to process the conditioner, if not, feel free to sit under a dryer or take a warm shower or bath. Finally rinse your hair and wrap in a towel, being sure not to rub or manipulate the braids.

Now it's time to apply a leave-in conditioner. You do not want to miss this step, especially if you have recently relaxed your hair. A leave-in conditioner aids in the continued strengthening of the hair, which hair needs while in extensions. Don't forget your last step, spraying a moisturizing braid spray on the braids daily. This will ensure the hair is being well moisturized while in the extensions.

This process keeps my hair healthy, strong and moisturized and minimizes the amount of hair on the floor during the dreaded braid extension take down. It is important to remember when taking down the extensions that you may have some lint balls that accumulate at the base of the braid. Do not comb the lint out, but carefully pick it out after taking down each braid.

Well, I like wearing a weave
(As long as you take care of it, that's fine)

Many of us yearn for long beautiful, healthy hair, but the damage over the years may have caused our hair to be short and brittle. If this is the case for you, a hair weave may be the answer. Weaves are NOT only used to cover up damaged hair, but can be used in order to transition from relaxed hair to natural hair; used to grow out a cut, temporarily protect the hair from the elements, or to minimize or eliminate combing, brushing and using heat on your own hair for long periods of time. Whatever the reason you may chose to wear a weave; a hair weave requires careful maintenance otherwise you may feel as if you wasted a lot of money and time and if you neglect your own hair and scalp while wearing a weave, you may end up with more damage than you began with. Here are 8 tips for maintaining a weave.

1. If you plan on wearing weave for an extended period of time, be sure to get quality hair, hair that can withstand washing and regular styling without getting too matted or ratty looking.

2. Be sure to comb through the hair regularly in order to avoid excessive tangling and matting. When combing the hair, start at the ends and comb

upward to the scalp. Use a semi-wide or wide tooth comb to avoid excessive stress on the hair.

3. Brush or comb the hair to cut down on tangles and massage the scalp to loosen up any build up before washing.

4. Washing the hair in the shower is much easier than in a sink. Be sure to use cool water on the hair and NOT hot. As the water is running through the hair, be sure to allow as much access as possible to the scalp. During the process finger comb the hair so that it remains as detangled as possible.

5. Instead of saturating the entire head with shampoo, focus on the scalp by massaging the shampoo carefully between the tracks.

6. Avoid using products that contain alcohol, mineral oils, and other harsh ingredients because it can greatly alter the quality of the weave including causing excessive dryness, matting and loss of shine.

7. Depending on the desired style, a weave can be wrapped at night in a satin scarf in the same way you regularly wrap your hair. It can be wrapped in a circle around the head, or maybe set with rollers, or pins;

however you decide to prepare it at night, the most important element is a satin scarf or pillowcase to avoid drying the hair out.

8. Do not over due it with the styling products as it can decrease the quality of the weave, although you should definitely use some form of moisturizer in order to keep your own hair moisturized and healthy.

If you follow these suggestions, a weave can be an awesome way of protecting and growing your own hair. Of course a professional is always the best way to go as they are skillfully trained and can help with the upkeep and maintenance of a weave, but if you are a do-it-yourselfer, I would suggest investing in a DVD that teaches techniques on weaving in order to be sure you are giving your hair the best care possible.

My Natural Story

Transitioning is the process of growing out chemically altered hair back to its natural state. For approximately 20 years, I chemically altered my hair starting with a Jherri Curl then later a relaxer. I have experienced pretty much every hairstyle except for locs, which I am hoping to experience in the near future. Black women in general experiment a lot with their hair and probably experience hundreds of hairstyles throughout their lifetime. Unfortunately most of us with a relaxer experienced our natural hair when we were too young to remember it or to deal with it on our own; therefore we have no idea how to handle the naps, kinks, coils and waves we have underneath our altered tresses.

If you recall the story about me losing my hair after a weaving incident, you know that I was devastated. I was told by a doctor that relaxing my hair could have contributed to the hair loss and that they see many Black women with issues like mines. It was explained to me that we have more scalp and hair loss concerns than any other race because we chemically alter our hair more often. We suffer more from traction alopecia, which is balding from pulling the hair too tightly in braids or in a ponytail, and traumatic or chemical alopecia which are caused primarily by relaxing the hair too often and/or incorrectly.

Despite being warned against continued chemical use, I could not bring myself to stop relaxing my hair. There was no way in the world I would be caught with a nappy head. So instead of completely stopping, I would relax around the bald spot as much as possible and only touch-up the new growth in the balding and thinning areas during every third application, at which time it would commence to break completely off. I did this for 10 years. In those 10 years, I was unable to grow healthy, long hair in certain areas of my head, although the rest of my hair flourished and was long and thick enough to disguise the thinning, damaged hair.

One day while looking for the miracle cure for the thinned areas, I came across an article that indicated that some cases of traumatic or chemical alopecia, which I ultimately decided I had, can be reversed if the trauma is stopped. This was the exact same thing the dermatologist told me 8 years prior, but I was hard headed and my mind could not fathom life without a relaxer. By this time in my life, my mind had witnessed and gone through more than I ever thought possible and I could pretty much fathom anything; going without a relaxer for a year was nothing. So, on December 30, 2004, I applied my last relaxer.

Because I was pretty talented in the hair styling department, I did some research on great transitioning styles I could do myself and planned a year's worth of styles; charting how long I would keep each style and how I would maintain it. This made it easier for me to stay on course and not feel so anxious when the time came to get rid of the old style and change to the new.

Approximately 6 weeks after my last relaxer, it was time to start the transitioning styles because I started to have a difficult time dealing with the two textures. My routine was going to be pretty simple; I would do roller-sets and cornrows for the first 6 months and extensions for the remainder of the year; in between each style, I would cut about an inch of hair off until all of the relaxer was gone and I could start over fresh telaxing my hair.

On August 25, 2005, I took down my second set of extensions and was ready to put my third set in. This time, instead of cutting off an inch, I decided to cut all of the relaxer out. Gradually, I was falling in love with the kinks and coils that I never had the opportunity to get to know, and I wanted to see them in all of their glory; without the straight ends attached. After I finished cutting it, I had a little afro and I, quite honestly, looked like a 14 year old boy. I was excited, anxious and kind of confused about my new found naps. I liked them, but not on me; I wanted to take them for a spin, but I wasn't sure what people would say or think; maybe if I put on some make-up and some really cute earrings, I would look good; maybe if I put some product in my hair, my naps might turn into curls; I decided that I was too unsure to try just yet, but I knew that I would have to do it soon because I couldn't keep my hands out of my new found head of hair.

So, after playing in my little afro for a while, I decided to put my extensions back in when I discovered my hair was too coily and too short to fit neatly in the extensions. I totally freaked out because I had no plan in place for this. I had to go to work in the morning and there was no way I was going to walk in that office where I am the only Black person with this itty bitty afro when I had just had braid extensions down my back the day before. I tried unsuccessfully for hours to get the extensions to go in neatly. I had my emergency relaxer stashed under my bathroom sink just for a moment like this. I would just telax it and wear a cute short style until it grew back. I was pretty sure I could manage something once my hair was straighter. Just as I went to mix the relaxer, I realized that I had just washed my hair and I couldn't relax it for another 48 hours at least. So, I decided to go to the internet and search for natural hair styles that I could manage with my hair's length and texture.

After hours of searching, I decided that finger coils would be the easiest and least time consuming, as well as the cutest style to do. It took me about 2.5 hours to complete and when I finished my hair was absolutely gorgeous; I looked so sophisticated. I was more than pleased with the outcome, I was downright ecstatic. I couldn't stop looking in the mirror because the person starring back did not look like me nor did she feel like me.

After I finished, I decided I probably should tell my boyfriend since he didn't know anything about my hair plans. He thought I was on a challenge to grow my hair as long as possible and that's why I was wearing extensions so much. At first I just told him that I cut it and he assumed I cut it into a bob or some other short style. When I told him that I had finger coils and that I no longer had a relaxer, he freaked out and said he was on his way over to see it.

While waiting for him to come, I was so nervous and worried that he wouldn't like it. I decided that if he didn't like it, I would just relax it and start over with my transitioning. Almost simultaneously another thought entered my mind, a stronger more confident thought decided that I didn't care if he liked it or not, I loved it and I was keeping it. That very moment I decided to never let anyone's opinion of me make me change who I am or what I think about myself; I instantly felt more confident and stronger; prouder and liberated. Fortunately, he saw it, fell in love with it, and now he's almost as obsessed with it as I am. The only regret that I have about going natural is not doing it sooner.

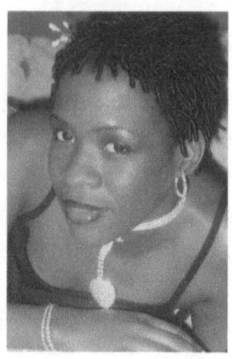

Actual Coils

Although I do love my natural hair and find myself more drawn to natural styles, I do understand the desire to want to relax our hair. I have very nappy and coily hair and it is not the easiest hair type to manage. I also have a lot of hair, thus making it that much more difficult to handle. I know what it is like to wash, condition, detangle and style unruly hair; it's not fun and it is very time consuming and not a lot of people have the time or patience it takes to get through this process. This is why I would never insist a person go natural because it really does take a lot of dedication.

Dealing with natural hair is so different then dealing with relaxed hair. We have to wash our hair differently, detangle it differently, comb it differently, use different styling products, and learn to style differently. I also noticed that the longer a person is natural, the more conscious we become of ingredients in products we put onto our hair, making a trip to the hair store becomes more like a trip to the grocery store with all the label reading. This consciousness of hair ingredient leads to a closer consciousness of the ingredients in the foods we put into our bodies; then leads to a consciousness of the ingredients we put into our minds. Not to mention the fact that most women become more patient, which dealing with natural hair takes a lot of. So, many women consider going natural a spiritual, mental and emotional transition as well as a physical one.

Washing and Conditioning Natural Tresses
(No, it's not the same as with a relaxer)

Depending on how long your natural hair is, there are a couple different ways to wash it effectively. Hair that is up to 4 inches can be washed pretty simply; wet the hair; add cleansing agent, gently massage the scalp and finger comb the hair as you are washing it to cut down on tangling. However, hair that is any longer than 4 inches may require a little more time and effort. The best way to begin is to separate the hair into 5-10 sections, depending on the length of the hair, by either putting them into ponytails or braids. Then wash each section separately, making sure to finger comb while washing to cut down on tangles.

I would also recommend no-pooing or co-washing, which just means you wash your hair with cheap conditioner instead of actual shampoo. This will allow the hair to retain moisture and avoid that stripped feeling we get after shampooing. Conditioners contain enough detergents to effectively cleanse the scalp, yet leaving enough oil to combat over drying. It also has a great "slippage" factor which helps with the detangling process. If you do decide to wash your hair this way, I would recommend incorporating a baking soda or apple cider vinegar (ACV) rinse after every few washes. This is used to clarify the scalp, which just means to make sure it gets a really thorough cleansing. You can also use a clarifying shampoo, but I would dilute it and add oil, and pour it over my scalp, in the same manner you would wash braid extensions, and then massage instead of using full strength. There are also clarifying conditioners you can use in place of clarifying shampoo. Below are the simple mixtures for the apple cider vinegar rinse and the baking soda rinse.

*2 cups of water, as cold as you can stand it and 10 teaspoons of ACV
*2 cups of warm water to 1 tablespoon of baking soda
Pour over the scalp, massage and then rinse. The ACV mixture does not have to be rinsed out as the smell will go away on its own.

Some people are not very comfortable with washing their hair and not having suds. If this is the case, I would definitely recommend you find a shampoo that does not contain sodium lauryl sulphate (SLS) or sodium laureth sulphate (SLES). Even with using these shampoos, it may be a good idea to add a squirt of castor oil or olive oil to every squirt of shampoo, just to reserve a certain level of moisture in the hair.

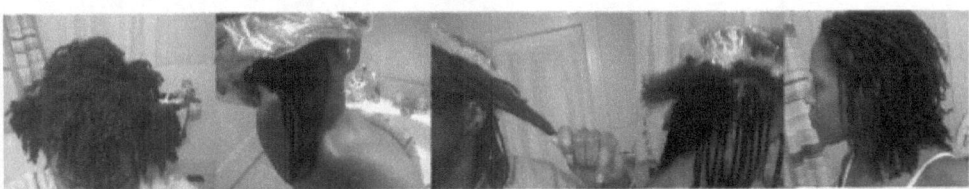

Dry Separate the hair 3-8 sections. Spray with Growth | Place the cap back on the hair | •Take out enough hair to do about 5-10 twist
•Take the Wisdom Moisturizer and disperse it through the section
•Hold the hair out and run the blow-dryer through the length of the hair (don't dry completely)This is just to stretch the hair for hanging twist (optional) | Continue this process throughout

Styling My Natural Tresses

I quickly learned that going natural meant no more long flowing hair. When I first saw my TWA (Teeny Weenie Afro), I must admit that I was quite shocked as I had no idea what I would do with it. I saw so many women rocking afros during my research that looked absolutely fabulous, but that was one style that I had a hard time accepting on myself. So, I decided that I needed to learn to do some other styles.

My first attempt at styling my natural hair was an overwhelming success. I had about 1.5 inches of hair and decided to do finger coils. This is one of the easiest natural styles to do. Essentially, finger coils are premature locs formed by twisting small portions of hair between the fingers or with a comb (the comb method is not so easy).

The finger coils were my signature style for the first 6 months of being natural. They were very easy to do and they looked good when I wore my office attire or when I was out for a night on the town. The style is both funky and sophisticated.

After about 6 months, my hair grew enough for me to be comfortable wearing other styles. I decided I would try what are called two-strand twists. Two strand twists resemble the kinky twist extensions. This style is also very easy. If you have ever done ponytails with twist and barrettes, you are doing two-strand twists. The only difference is there is no ponytail and more than likely the twist are much smaller. For those who have never had the pleasure of twisting, all you have to do is take two evenly sized strands of hair and wrap them around each other; starting at the scalp and moving down until you reach the end.

When you unravel two-strand twist or the coils an entire new look is created. Unraveled two-strand twists are called twist outs and, you guessed it; the unraveled coils is called a coil-out. For the two years I have been natural I have worn my hair in hundreds of variations of the coils, coil-outs, two strand twist, and two strand twist-outs.

I know that having healthy hair seems like a lot of drama, but really it isn't. Once you get your own routine and hair regimen together, it really is rather simple. Although this book has a lot of information there really is a somewhat simple equation to follow and you are well on your way to beautiful black healthy hair; Washing (water) + Deep Conditioning (protein) + Moisturizing = BBHH (Beautiful, Black, Health, Hair)

Pick Your Hair Care Products Wisely
(They may end up somewhere other than your hair)

Many of the ingredients in our hair care products and other personal care products are toxic. Our skin is the largest organ. Toxins are absorbed very quickly through our skin and enter into our blood stream quicker than the nutrients from the foods we eat. The level of toxicity in the ingredients in personal care products are not regulated, therefore a company could produce a product that contains 100% of an ingredient that is considered toxic, such as baby oil, which is 100% mineral oil.

A couple of years ago I begin using henna to dye my hair. Henna is a leaf that is essentially crushed into a powder. When it is mixed with an acid such as vinegar or the acid from a citrus fruit, it releases a dye that can be used for the hair. Because leaves are green, the mixture is green as well. After the process, I went to the restroom was alarmed when I noticed that my urine was bright green. This incident made me realize just how much our skin absorbs in a short amount of time. Just think about the toxins we are absorbing when we "grease" our scalps with mineral oil based hair care products.

Many products advertise the use of vitamins, oils and butters as ingredients in their products, but when you read the labels, the ingredient is listed very close to the bottom of the label. This means there is a very small amount of the ingredient in the product and more likely than not, it is not enough to be very effective. So, regardless if the label reads "now with vitamins" or "Shea butter formula", or "Olive oil properties", be sure to check the ingredients on the label to see how close to the top of the label the ingredient actually falls.

For 12 years I looked for hair care products that not only stated they were geared towards African American hair, but that actually contained ingredients that proved they were for African American hair and contained ingredients that were safe for use. I found this task to be daunting; therefore I formulated my own healthy hair care products that cleanse, strengthens and moisturizes Black hair. My products along with this guide will allow you to grow your hair to its fullest potential while permitting you to avoid the unhealthy toxins that are in the majority of hair care products.

Sweet Nature by Eddie Healthy Hair Care Products

"Inspiration" Moisturizing Shampoo: No lauryl sulphate (SLS) & sodium laureth sulphate (SLES). This shampoo will leave your hair clean, but not stripped of all its natural oils. It is infused with 6-blended, nutrient rich carrier oils and raw honey. This will not only leave the hair feeling clean, but it will also leave your scalp healthier.

"Love" Stimulating Deep Conditioner: Detangling will be a breeze with this rich and creamy conditioner. The tingling sensation of the peppermint oil will awaken your scalp and stimulate and enrich your follicles and the nutrient rich oils and honey will provide the needed vitamins for a healthy, happy scalp.

"Growth" Daily Moisturizing Detangling Spray: This is a multi-purpose spray, used as a detangler, braid spray, scalp energizer, and moisturizer. It will not only leave the hair quenched, soft and unbelievably manageable, but aloe vera, which is the base of the spray, will assist in healthy blood flow while delivering nutrients to the follicles. Spray your hair daily and bask in the softness.

"Dream" Cream Moisturizer: This moisturizer is made with Shea Butter, Olive Butter, Cocoa Butter and other lovely, moisturizing butter as well as nutrient rich carrier oils and aloe vera. It will leave your hair super soft and ultra moisturized. This moisturizer is best used on people with coily to curly hair. Its creamy consistency is lighter, yet "wetter" than Wisdom.

"Wisdom" Shea-Cocoa Moisturizer: Wisdom Shea-Cocoa Butter is Shea butter and cocoa butter based moisturizer that contains many other oils and butters. The moisturizer is thick and rich and give the hair a slight hold, which is excellent to replace gel or using while braiding or two-strand twisting.

Sprit Follicle Stimulator: Is sulfur based and contains oils and herbs that block DHT and that carry nutrients directly to the follicle, while delivering needed soothing and healing properties to the scalp. The combination of the herbs, sulfur and oils, allows the hair to grow healthier, stronger hair, longer hair faster! You won't BELIEBVE the growth!

Sweet Nature by Eddie Silk Amino Protein Mask: it is infused with some of the same goodness as the Love Deep Conditioner, but contains a bit more protein to help reinforce the hair's strength, it also has twice the amount of honey and I have substituted the peppermint EO with lavender

EO. Lavender disinfects the scalp, enhances blood circulation, treats scalp psoriasis, soothes the scalp and works to fight hair loss such as alopecia areata. Honey is also excellent for hair loss and increases the health of your hair follicles and your scalp at the same time. Not only will your hair be stronger and healthier, but so soft and super manageable.

Sweet Nature Vitamins Today, most all women and men are not giving their hair what it needs to grow healthy, shiny and vibrant. My vitamins rejuvenate your hair growth by feeding your hair all the natural amino acids, minerals, vitamin, protein and overall nutrition needed for your hair to reach its fullest potential! All natural and easy to swallow hair vitamins! Great for skin and fingernails also!

Journey Hair Milk: This moisturizer is super light weight, yet very rich. It will leave the hair ultra moisturized and soft with no sticky or heavy feeling like some hair milk. This cherry-vanilla scented moisturizer is also made with a Shea butter based and infused with aloe vera and several other nutrient rich ingredients.

Vitamins for healthy hair growth

Vitamin	Hair Function	Food Source	Recommended Dosage
A	Antioxidant that helps produce healthy sebum in the scalp	Fish liver oil, meat, milk, cheese, eggs, spinach, broccoli, cabbage, carrots, apricots, pumpkins and peaches,	5,000 IU *More than 25,000 IU daily is toxic and can cause hair loss and other serious health problems
B1 (Thiamin)	Healthy hair growth	Green veggies, corn, potatoes, oats, rice, plums, raisins, nuts, yeast, ham	RDI 1.5 mg/RDA1.5mg
B2 (Riboflavin)	Prevents dandruff	Liver, cheese, milk, eggs, avocado, green/yellow veggies, grains, nuts	RDI 1.7 mg/RDA1.7mg
B3 (Niacin)	Promotes scalp circulation	Brewer's yeast, wheat germ, fish, chicken, turkey and meat	15 mg *Taking more than 25 mg a day can result in "niacin flush" - a temporary heat sensation due to blood cell dilatation
B5 (Pantothenic Acid)	Prevents graying and hair loss	Whole grain cereals, brewer's yeast, organ meats and egg yolks	4-7 mg
B12	Prevents hair loss	Beef, liver, egg yolks, crab, clams, sardines, salmon, oysters, herring, chicken, milk	2 mg
C	Antioxidant that helps maintain skin & hair health.	Citrus fruits, strawberries, kiwi, cantaloupe, pineapple, tomatoes, green peppers, potatoes and dark green vegetables	60 mg
E	Antioxidant that enhances scalp circulation	Cold-pressed vegetable oils, wheat germ oil, soybeans, raw seeds and nuts, dried beans, and leafy green vegetables	Up to 400 *Can raise blood pressure and reduce blood clotting.

Minerals for healthy hair growth

Mineral	Hair Function	Food Source	Recommended Dosage
Calcium	Essential for healthy hair growth	Dairy, tofu, fish, nuts, brewer's yeast, beans, lentils and sesame seeds	Up to 1,500 mg *Too much calcium can inhibit the absorption of zinc and iron
Chromium	Helps prevent hyperglycemia and hypoglycemia, both of which can cause hair loss	Brewer's yeast, liver, beef and whole wheat bread	Up to 120 mg *who are allergic to yeast should not take chromium supplements
Copper	Helps prevent hair loss. Assist with keep original hair color	Shellfish, liver, green vegetables, whole grains, eggs, chicken, beans, nuts	Up to 3 mg *High levels can lead to dry hair, hair loss
Iodine	Helps regulate thyroid hormones and prevents dry hair and hair loss	Fish, seaweed, kelp, iodized salt, garlic, mushrooms, cheese	150 mcg
Iron	Prevents hair loss	Liver, eggs, fish, chicken, whole grains, green vegetables and dried fruits	15 mg *much can lead to malfunctions of the liver and spleen
Magnesium	Works with calcium to promote healthy hair growth	Green vegetables, wheat germ, whole grains, nuts, soy beans, chickpeas and fish	280 mg
Manganese	Prevents slow hair growth	Whole grain cereals, eggs, avocados, nuts, seeds, beans, peas, fish, meat and chicken	3-9 mg
Potassium	Regulates circulation and promotes healthy hair growth	bananas, lima beans, brown rice, dates, figs, dried fruit, garlic, nuts, potatoes, raisins, yams and yogurt.	3,500 mg.
Selenium	Strengthen hair & Keeps skin and scalp supple and elastic	yeast, meat, fish, grains, tuna and broccoli	55 mcg *excess of Selenium can be toxic, leading to the loss of hair, nails and teeth
Silica	Strengthens hair and prevents hair loss	Seafood, rice, soybeans, green vegetables	55 mcg

Sulfur or MSM	main component to hair's structure	Onions, garlic, eggs, asparagus, meat, fish and dairy products	1-3 g
Zinc	A deficiency can lead to dry hair and oily skin	Spinach, sunflower seeds, mushrooms, whole grains, red meat and brewer's yeast	12 mg *Too much can interfere with iron absorption

Homemade Deep Conditioners

1 small jar of real mayonnaise
1/2 of an avocado
Mix with your hands or with a hand held mixer in a medium bowl. After applying to towel dried hair, place a shower cap on the hair. For a more deep conditioning apply a hot towel around the cap; let sit for 20 minutes then rinse. You can also do a deep conditioning with mayonnaise by itself. Just remember to use real mayonnaise and not salad dressing.

1 avocado
1 can coconut milk
Mash avocado and slowly add coconut milk until smooth and the consistency of hair conditioner. Work through hair to ends. Rinse after 15 minutes then shampoo

1 teaspoon baby oil
1 egg yolk
1 cup water
Beat the egg yolk until it's frothy, add the oil then beat again. Add to the water. Massage into the scalp and throughout your hair. Rinse well

1/2 a banana,
1/4 avocado,
1/4 cantaloupe,
1 tablespoon wheat germ oil and
1 tablespoon plain yogurt.
For extra conditioning, squeeze in the contents of a vitamin E capsule. Leave in hair for 15 minutes.
Combine all ingredients in a medium bowl and mix with hand held mixer. Continue until mix is slightly thicker than yogurt. Apply to towel dried hair. Rinse well.

1 cup plain yogurt
2 tablespoon honey
1 teaspoon vegetable glycerin
 Combine all ingredients in a medium bowl and stir with spoon. Apply to towel dried hair. Work up body heat by exercising or taking a warm bath or shower. Rinse well.

½ cup plain yogurt
1 egg white
Beat the egg until frothy then add it to the yogurt. Leave on for about 15 minutes, making sure to process with a plastic bag. Rinse

4 teaspoons of honey
¼ cup of extra virgin olive oil
Warm honey either in hot water or in the microwave (be extremely careful using the microwave). Add the olive oil and apply to hair. Process with a plastic bag for 15-30 minutes. Rinse.

Tips

Diluting some products make them last longer, and don't compromise their effectiveness. Try diluting your shampoo by pouring the desired amount into a large cup and then filling the cup with water. Pour the shampoo over your scalp and massage for a few minutes. This will give you a thoroughly cleansed scalp using less shampoo. Also try diluting your leave-in conditioners. Most leave-ins are made primarily of water and can actually stand to be diluted a little more. Below are quick instructions on how to dilute your leave-in conditioner:

Leave in conditioner spritz
Empty 4 oz spray bottle
2 oz liquid leave-in conditioner or setting lotion
2 oz distilled water (boiled)
5 drops of peppermint oil
5 drops of rosemary oil

Add drops of peppermint oil to the majority of your products. Peppermint oil provides that tingling sensation that stimulates the scalp. Just remember that essential oils are very concentrated and a little goes a long way. Try adding only 3-5 drops to every 4 oz of product.

Add natural ingredients to commercial products. Sometimes it is really expensive and may seem wasteful to make a hair smoothie out of food you could eat. This is why I rarely use 100% food ingredients. What I do is add a food item or two to my store bought conditioners. I generally deep condition my hair with the cholesterol deep conditioner; no particular brand, whatever is least expensive because I plan to doctor it up anyhow. I add either of these in different combinations, depending on what I have on hand or what I think my hair really needs, of the following ingredients: honey, avocado, plain yogurt, olive oil, real mayonnaise, castor oil, coconut oil, or coconut milk. All of these ingredients can be mixed with conditioners or when two or more are mixed together, to make a homemade conditioner. The olive oil, castor oil and coconut oil can be mixed with your hair products to aid in additional moisture as well.

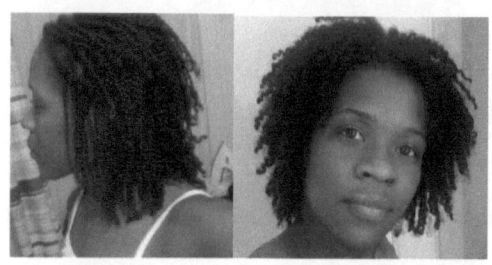

Instructions for 2-Strand Twists

- Place hair in 5-10 sections by using braids or puffs. If your hair is shorter than 4 inches, skip the sectioning part.

- Wash each section separately and replace in a braid or puff. Continue this until all sections are complete.

- Apply deep conditioner to each section and replace in a braid or puff

- Put on a plastic shower cap and either sit under a dryer or work up some body heat by exercising, taking a warm shower, or just doing some work around the house for 15-30 minutes.

- Rinse each section separately and replace in a braid or puff

- Spray on a leave-in conditioner and replace in a braid or puff

- Replace plastic cap over entire head and take out one section at a time

- Towel blot, apply product and then blow dry on lowest setting, while stretching hair outwards. Dry only about 80%.

- Depending on the desired size of your twist, take two equal sections and twist them around each other.

Instructions for Coils

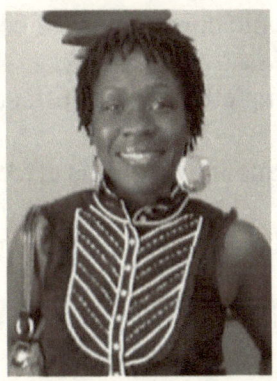

- Place hair in 5-10 sections by using braids or puffs. If your hair is shorter than 4 inches, skip the sectioning part.

- Wash each section separately and replace in a braid or puff

- Deep condition each section and replace in a braid or puff

- Spray on a leave in conditioner and replace in a braid or puff

- Towel dry hair, then apply product. Product should be a heavier cream like a Shea butter consistency.

- Depending on how large you like your coils, take the desired sized section of hair, then begin to roll it in between your index finger and thumb, starting at the root and twisting downward.

To do a coil-out separate each coil into 2-3 sections, being careful to twist/roll each section in the direction of the original coil while separating

Ingredient Glossary

1,4-Dioxane - A carcinogenic contaminant of cosmetic products. Almost 50% of cosmetics containing ethoxylated surfactants were found to contain dioxane. 1,4-Dioxane may exert its effects through inhalation, skin absorption and ingestion. It is listed as a carcinogen. Dioxane is an eye and mucous membrane irritant, primary skin irritant, central nervous system depressant. Acute exposure can cause headaches, dizziness and narcosis. Chronic inhalation exposure can cause damage to internal organs and cause blood disorders.

DEA (diet hanolamine) MEA (monoethanolamine) TEA (triethanolamine) - Used in cosmetics to adjust the pH, and used with many fatty acids to convert acid to salt (stearate), which then becomes the base for a cleanser. TEA causes allergic reactions including eye problems, dryness of hair and skin, and could be toxic if absorbed into the body over a long period of time. These chemicals are already restricted in Europe due to known carcinogenic effects.

FD&C Color Pigments – Synthetic colors made from coal tar. Contain heavy metal salts that deposit toxins onto the skin, causing skin sensitivity and irritation. Animal studies have shown almost all of them to be carcinogenic.

Fragrance - Fragrance on a label can indicate the presence of up to four thousand separate ingredients, many toxic or carcinogenic. Symptoms reported to the USA FDA include headaches, dizziness, allergic rashes, skin discoloration, violent coughing and vomiting, and skin irritation. Clinical observation proves fragrances can affect the central nervous system, causing depression, hyperactivity, and irritability

Imidazolidinyl Urea and DMDM Hydantoin:

These are two of the many preservatives that release formaldehyde According to the Mayo Clinic, formaldehyde can irritate the respiratory system, cause skin reactions and trigger heart palpitations. Exposure to formaldehyde may cause joint pain, allergies, depression, headaches, chest pains, ear infections, chronic fatigue, dizziness and loss of sleep. It can also aggravate coughs and colds and trigger asthma. Serious side effects include weakening of the immune system and cancer. Nearly all brands of skin, body and hair care, antiperspirants and nail polish found in stores contain formaldehyde-releasing ingredients.

Mineral Oil - Petroleum by-product that coats the skin like plastic, clogging the pores. Interferes with skin's ability to eliminate toxins, promoting acne and other disorders. Slows down skin function and cell development, resulting in premature aging. Used in many products (baby oil is 100% mineral oil!) Any mineral oil derivative can be contaminated with cancer causing PAH's (Polycyclic Aromatic Hydrocarbons). Manufacturers use petroleum because it is unbelievably cheap.

Polyethylene Glycol (PEG) - Potentially carcinogenic petroleum ingredient that can alter and reduce the skin's natural moisture factor. This could increase the appearance of aging and leave you more vulnerable to bacteria. Used in cleansers to dissolve oil and grease. It adjusts the melting point and thickens products. Also used in caustic spray-on oven cleaners.

Propylene Glycol (PG) - Propylene glycol (PG) is a petroleum derivative. It penetrates the skin and can weaken protein and cellular structure. The EPA considers PG so toxic that it requires workers to wear protective gloves, clothing and goggles and to dispose of any PG solutions by burying them in the ground. Because PG penetrates the skin so quickly, the EPA warns against skin contact to prevent consequences such as brain, liver, and kidney abnormalities.

Sodium Lauryl Sulfate (SLS) and Lauryl Sulfate (SLS) and Sodium Laureth Sulfate (SLES) and Ammonium Lauryl Sulfate (ALS) - Used in car washes, garage floor cleaners and engine degreasers - and in 90% of products that foam. Animals exposed to SLS and ALS experience eye damage, central nervous system depression, labored breathing, diarrhea,

3

severe skin irritation, and even death. Young eyes may not develop

properly if exposed to SLS and ALS because proteins are dissolved. SLS

and ALS may also damage the skin's immune system by causing layers to

separate and inflame. It is frequently disguised in semi-natural cosmetics

with the explanation